BRAIN WASH RECIPES

A 10-DAY brain wash diet plan to help shape your cognitive health and make you cultivate a more purposeful and fulfilling life.

By

Kim Cox

Copyright © 2020, By: *Kim Cox*

ISBN: 978-1-950772-79-7

All Rights Reserved. No part of this publication may be reproduced in any form or by any means, including scanning, photocopying, or otherwise without prior written permission of the copyright holder.

Disclaimer:

The information provided in this book is designed to provide helpful information on the subjects discussed. The publisher and author are not responsible for any specific health or allergy needs that may require medical supervision and are not liable for any damages or negative consequences from any treatment, action, application or preparation, to any person reading or following the information in this book.

Table of Contents

INTRODUCTION 6
   BRAIN WASH 6

The Brain Wash Recipes 9
   Finding Connection in the Kitchen 9

BASICS 9
   Vegetable Stock 9
   Leize's Basic Vinaigrette 14
   Aioli 16
   Brain Wash Dry Rub for Meats, Poultry, and Fish ... 20
   Ricotta Cheese 23
   Stone Age Bread 26

DELECTABLE BRAIN WASH RECIPE FOR BREAKFAST 29
   All-in-One Breakfast 29
   Almost Muesli 31
   Avocado Toast 33
   Breakfast Crepes 37
   Greens with Eggs 41
   Cauliflower Pancakes 44

DELECTABLE BRAIN WASH APPETIZERS, SOUPS, SALADS, AND SMALL PLATES 48
   Cauliflower Hummus 48
   Madras Pea Soup 51
   Garlic Soup 56
   Chicken Caesar Salad 60
   Chicory Salad with Tahini Dressing 65

Directions for the Tahini Dressing: 66

Sesame Beef Kebabs with Avocado Dipping Sauce 68

Avocado Dipping Sauce 72

Grilled Clams with Citrus-Herb Sauce 73

Citrus-Herb Sauce 75

DELECTABLE BRAIN WASH ENTRÉES 77

Lamb with Mustard Sauce 77

Deviled Cornish Game Hens 79

Almost Tandoori Chicken 82

Whole Roasted Striped Bass 86

Salmon with Green Sauce 90

Whole Roasted Salmon with Sunchokes and Leeks 93

Vegetable Lasagna 96

Grilled Cauliflower and Broccoli Steaks with Eggplant 101

DELECTABLE BRAIN WASH SIDES 106

Jicama Slaw 106

Sautéed Asparagus 108

Zucchini and Parsnip Noodles with Celery Root in Broccoli Sauce 110

Sunchoke Gratin 113

Leeks and Swiss Chard with Coconut Milk 116

Broccoli with Shallots and Red Pepper 119

Dandelion Greens with Onions 122

DELECTABLE BRAIN WASH DESSERTS 126

Favorite Chocolate Cake 126

Chocolate Chip Cookies 130

BRAIN WASH RECIPES

Almond-Coconut Biscotti 133
Ricotta Mousse 136
Almond Panna Cotta 138
DRINKS 141
Matcha Smoothie 141
Afternoon Pick-Me-Up 143
Hibiscus Tea 145
Gingerade 148
Powerhouse Coffee 150
Turmeric Milk Shake 152

INTRODUCTION

BRAIN WASH

Millions of people suffer today and do not realize or do not know what to do about it. However, some have given up and are going through the daily motions the best they can; it does not have to be this way.

Struggles, disappointments and challenges are inevitable, what is not inevitable is to feel chronically unleashed, foggy-minded, anxious for an uncertain and frustrated future, perhaps even shattered, for life itself.

We can eat what we want when we want. We can immerse ourselves completely in the vast and attractive world of digital media. We can buy goods and services and even find possible partners at the touch of a button or swipe a finger. We can live 24 hours in a virtual world in which everything about us is public. We struggle with the high rates of largely preventable diseases, and many of us are lonelier, depressed and anxious than ever.

It is difficult to consider this level of calm and satisfaction when the obligations of the modern world feel more inescapable and overwhelming with each passing day. But this may be your reality. The secret is to know what is happening in your head and then change the circuits that take you along destructive paths. This book is based on a simple premise:

Few people would debate the fact that bad decisions in our daily activities influence our health. Our dietary options are among many lifestyle habits that can lead to well-being or chronic diseases. Our mood and perceptions also directly and powerfully influence your dietary choices. In addition, this fact is exploited by the food production industry and creates a vicious circle that will destroy your health and your mind. In fact, we will show you how to break it. But this is much bigger than our food choices.

Billions of dollars are spent to convince us to keep looking for happiness the wrong way, literally reconnecting our brain so that we crave things that move us away from our goal. Moreover, this depressing scenario is now the norm, fueling a culture of chronic stress. Unfortunately, this type of stress is toxic to the brain, damaging the parts that help you have a sense of agency: feel in control of your life. And in your attempts to cope, you again use instant gratification, which makes it difficult to break the neural circuits that trigger and reinforce this behavior.

The Brain Wash Recipes

Finding Connection in the Kitchen

Food is a gateway for remodeling your brain and body. It is a ticket to a life of vibrant health and wellbeing. We've crafted original, deeply satisfying recipes that follow the Brain Wash protocol, including basics; breakfast dishes; appetizers, soups, salads, and small plates; sides, entrées, desserts, and drinks. These delicious anti-inflammatory menu options will fuel your body with the information it needs to optimize its overall function—supporting everything from the microbes in your gut to the neurons in your brain.

BASICS

Vegetable Stock

Makes about 6 cups
Time: 1 hour

Tips:

1. Remember, that there is nothing better than a nice, clean homemade broth or stock, even though you can buy fine quality preparations at the store.
2. Feel free add and/or subtract any vegetables you want, but remember that strongly flavored vegetables, such as cabbage and broccoli, will add bold flavor to the finished product. (NOTE: I always add a piece of ginger for its healing properties).

Ingredients:

3 large organic leeks, including some green parts (trimmed, well washed, and chopped)

2 cloves of organic garlic (peeled and chopped)

2 cups of chopped fresh organic mushrooms

2 organic bay leaves

Fine sea salt (to taste)

3 medium organic onions (peeled and chopped)

2 organic carrots (peeled, trimmed, and chopped)

1 organic fennel bulb (trimmed and chopped)

3–6 sprigs organic parsley

1-inch piece organic ginger (peeled)

1 teaspoon of organic black peppercorns

Directions:

1. First, combine the leeks, garlic, fennel, onions, carrots, and mushrooms in a large deep saucepan.
2. After which you add 7 cups water and stir to blend.
3. After that, add the bay leaves, ginger, parsley, and peppercorns along with the salt.
4. Then, place over high heat and bring to a boil.
5. At this point, cover and lower the heat to a gentle simmer.
6. This is when you simmer for 30 minutes, or until the liquid is nicely flavored by the vegetables.
7. Furthermore, remove from the heat and strain through a fine-mesh strainer into a clean container.

8. Finally, use immediately or let cool and store, covered, in the refrigerator for up to three days or in the freezer for up to three months.

VARIATIONS: Directions to make mushroom stock

First, add 7 ounces of dried mushrooms to the above recipe along with the onions and other vegetables and simmer for about 45 minutes, or until the stock has a distinct mushroom flavor. (NOTE: strain and store as directed).

Directions to make poultry or meat stock

1. First, roast the backs and wings of pasture-raised chicken or turkey at about 350°F for about 30 minutes, or until nicely browned.
2. On the other hand, roast the bones and a bit of stew meat from grass-fed animals at the same temperature for about 40 minutes, or until nicely browned.

3. Then, add the browned chicken or meat to the above recipe along with the herbs and proceed as directed.

Leize's Basic Vinaigrette

Makes about 2 cups
Preparation Time: About 15 minutes
Tip:
This recipe can also be made using avocado, coconut, or other nut oils.

Ingredients:

1½ teaspoons of organic Dijon mustard

About 1 tablespoon of chopped fresh organic herbs, such as basil, tarragon, parsley, or chives (optional)

2 tablespoons of organic red or better still white wine vinegar

Directions:

1. First, combine the vinegar, garlic, and salt in a small bowl.
2. After which you set aside to mellow for about 10 minutes.
3. Then, using a whisk, beat in the mustard, then slowly pour in the oil, a bit at a time,

whisking to emulsify. (**NOTE:** You may not need all the oil, depending upon how acidic you like your salad dressing).

4. After that, taste and season with additional salt, if necessary, and freshly ground black pepper. (**NOTE:** If using herbs, I suggest you whisk them in just before serving).
5. Finally, store in the refrigerator, bring to room temperature, and shake to blend before using.

VARIATIONS:

1. First, add 1 small peeled and minced shallot along with the mustard.
2. It you want to make balsamic vinaigrette; I suggest you replace the organic red or white wine vinegar with organic balsamic vinegar.

Aioli

Makes about 2 cups
Preparation Time: About 12 minutes
Ingredients:

1 tablespoon of organic champagne vinegar or better still freshly squeezed organic lemon juice

1 teaspoon of smashed organic garlic

1½–2 cups of organic extra virgin olive oil or better still avocado oil

2–3 threads saffron

3 large egg yolks from pasture-raised chickens, at room temperature

½ teaspoon of fine sea salt

¼ teaspoon of organic dry mustard powder

Directions:

1. First, place the saffron in the vinegar and let it infuse for at least 30 minutes.
2. Then, when ready to prepare the mayonnaise, fill the glass jar of a blender with boiling water and set it aside for a

couple of minutes. (NOTE: The idea is to heat the jar to help the egg yolks thicken).
3. After which you pour out the water and quickly wipe the jar dry.
4. After that, add the egg yolks and blend on medium speed until very thick.
5. At this point, add the garlic along with the salt and mustard and quickly incorporate.
6. This is when you add the vinegar and process to blend. (NOTE: You can either remove the saffron threads or leave them in. If left in, they will add a distinct yellow color to the finished product.)
7. Furthermore, with the motor running, begin adding the oil in an excruciatingly slow drip. (NOTE: the slower the drip, the more even the emulsion. When about half the oil has been added, you should have a sauce with the consistency of old-fashioned heavy cream, and you can begin adding the oil just a bit more quickly, because curdling will no longer be an issue. If the mixture seems too

thick—you want a soft, creamy mix—add just a smidgen more vinegar)
8. After that, continue adding oil until all of it has been absorbed into the
9. eggs.
10. In addition, if necessary, add just enough hot water to smooth the mix, usually no more than a scant tablespoon.
11. Then, scrape the aioli into a clean container with a lid.
12. Finally, cover and refrigerate for up to five days.

VARIATIONS:

1. First, stir in 2 tablespoons chopped fresh herbs, minced green or red hot chili peppers, grated horseradish, grated ginger, or minced bell peppers to the finished aioli.
2. After which you ground spices can also vary the flavor—cumin, cayenne pepper, and

cracked black pepper are favorite additions. NOTE: turmeric
3. and curry powder can give it a South Asian kick.

If you want to make avocado aioli:

First, add ½ cup mashed organic avocado along with the mustard and replace the champagne vinegar or lemon juice with freshly squeezed organic lime juice.

Brain Wash Dry Rub for Meats, Poultry, and Fish

Makes about 2 cups
Preparation Time: About 15 minutes
Tips:

1. This recipe is a terrific way to introduce our favorite good-for-you spices into everyday cooking.
2. Remember, it is quite potent but adds just the right amount of zest to pasture-raised poultry, grass-fed meats, or fatty wild fish such as salmon, particularly when grilled or roasted.

Ingredients:

3 whole organic star anise
2-inch piece dried organic ginger root
¼ cup of organic cumin seeds
1 tablespoon of whole organic allspice
1 teaspoon of dried organic crushed red pepper flakes (it is optional)
8 organic cardamom pods

3 (2-inch) organic cinnamon sticks

½ cup of organic coriander seeds

¼ cup of organic black or better still white peppercorns

1 teaspoon of whole organic cloves

Directions:

1. First, combine the star anise, ginger root, cardamom, cinnamon sticks, coriander and cumin seeds, peppercorns, allspice, and cloves in a medium frying pan over medium-low heat.
2. After which you cook, stirring frequently and/or shaking the pan, for about 3 minutes, or until the spices are very fragrant and starting to color.

NOTE: it is important to keep the spices moving in the pan so they don't burn.

3. After that, remove from the heat and set aside to cool to room temperature.
4. Then, when cool, place in a spice grinder, food processor, or blender and process to a smooth powder.

NOTE: if using, I suggest you add the crushed red pepper.

5. Finally, transfer to a glass container, cover, and store in a cool dark spot for up to six weeks.

Remember, dried ginger root is available at specialty food stores, health food stores, Asian markets, and online.

Ricotta Cheese

Makes about 1½ cups

Preparation Time: About 2¼ hours

Tips:

1. This recipe can be eaten as a dessert, breakfast treat, or added to many dishes for extra creaminess and stability.
2. It can also serve as a spread or as a component in salads. If you want to use it solely as a dessert, I suggest you add a teaspoon or so of stevia when you heat the milk.

Ingredients:

1 cup of organic heavy cream from grass-fed animals

1½ tablespoons of strained freshly squeezed organic lemon juice

2 cups of organic whole milk from grass-fed animals

½ teaspoon of fine sea salt (it is optional)

1 teaspoon of granulated organic stevia, or more to taste (it is optional)

Directions:

1. First, line the interior of a fine-mesh sieve with two layers of damp cheesecloth. **NOTE:** make sure you use pieces that are big enough to hang slightly over the edges of the sieve so that the mesh is completely covered.
2. After which you set the lined sieve on top of a nonreactive container, such as a glass or stainless steel bowl, large enough to allow a few inches of space between the bottom of the sieve and the bottom of the bowl; set aside.
3. After that, combine the milk and cream and, if using, the salt or stevia in a heavy-bottom saucepan over medium heat.
4. At this point, bring to a gentle boil and boil for 1 minute.
5. This is when you remove from the heat and stir in the lemon juice.

6. Furthermore, set aside to rest for about 4 minutes, or just until the mixture separates into visible curds.
7. After that, pour into the lined strainer, cover with plastic wrap, and set aside to allow the whey to drain for about 2 hours, or until the curds reach the desired consistency. NOTE: The longer you allow the mixture to drain, the denser the finished cheese. Do not discard the whey; it may be used as a beverage or in any recipe requiring it.
8. Then, remove the plastic wrap, scrape the ricotta from the cheesecloth, and place it in a nonreactive container.
9. Finally, store, covered, in the refrigerator for up to five days.

Stone Age Bread

Makes 1 loaf
Preparation Time: About 1½ hours
Tips:

1. This recipe is easy to make, exceedingly nutritious, a great alternative to white bread, and very filling.
2. In this recipe you do not need to chop the seeds and nuts; use them whole, just as they are.

Ingredients

3½ ounces of raw unsalted organic sunflower seeds

3½ ounces of organic sesame seeds

3½ ounces of raw unsalted organic walnut pieces

2 teaspoons of fine sea salt

3½ ounces of raw unsalted organic pumpkin seeds

3½ ounces of raw unsalted organic flaxseeds

3½ ounces of raw unsalted organic almond slivers
5 large organic eggs from pasture-raised chickens, at room temperature, lightly beaten
½ cup of organic extra virgin olive oil

Directions:

1. Meanwhile, heat the oven to 325°F.
2. After which you butter a 9 × 5 × 3-inch loaf pan and line the bottom with parchment paper cut to fit.
3. After that, butter the top of the parchment paper.
4. Then, combine all the seeds and nuts in a large mixing bowl.
5. At this point, add the eggs, olive oil, and salt and stir to combine completely.
6. This is when you scrape the mixture into the prepared loaf pan.
7. Furthermore, transfer to the preheated oven and bake for about 1 hour, or until firm.
8. After that, remove the pan from the oven and let rest for 15 minutes.

9. In addition, turn the pan upside down and tap the bread out onto a cooling rack.
10. Finally, allow to cool slightly before cutting.
11. Make sure you store in an airtight container in the refrigerator.

DELECTABLE BRAIN WASH RECIPE FOR BREAKFAST

All-in-One Breakfast

Serves 2

Preparation Time: About 7 minutes

Tips:

1. This recipe is easy and quick—and such a healthful breakfast.
2. Remember, the greens, the ginger, the avocado, and the turmeric give you all you need to get your day started on the right note.

Ingredients:

1 large organic avocado (peeled and pitted)

1 cup of organic baby spinach leaves

½ teaspoon of grated organic ginger

2 cups of organic coconut water

4 sprigs organic flat-leaf parsley

1 large leaf organic kale, trimmed of its tough stalk and chopped

2 tablespoons of organic mint leaves

¼ teaspoon of organic ground turmeric

Directions:

1. First, combine the avocado, spinach, ginger, parsley, kale, mint, and turmeric in a blender.
2. After which you add the coconut water and 4 ice cubes and process to a smooth puree.
3. Then, pour into two chilled glasses and drink up!

Almost Muesli

Serves 2
Preparation Time: About 5 minutes
Tip:
This recipe has a bit more heft than the usual muesli and gives a warming welcome to a chilly morning and it is about as healthful a breakfast as we can imagine to start your day.

Ingredients:
½ cup of organic hemp seeds
¼ cup of organic oat flakes
1 tablespoon of raw unsalted organic flaxseeds
⅛ teaspoon of organic ground ginger
½ cup of organic blueberries
½ cup of chopped raw unsalted organic almonds
½ cup of unsweetened flaked organic coconut
2 tablespoons of raw unsalted organic chia seeds
¼ teaspoon of organic ground cinnamon
1½ cups of unsweetened organic coconut milk
1 teaspoon of MCT oil

Directions:

1. First, combine the hemp seeds, oats, flaxseeds, cinnamon, almonds, coconut, chia seeds, and ginger in a small saucepan.
2. After which you stir in the coconut milk and oil and place over medium heat.
3. After that, bring to a simmer and cook, stirring, for a couple of minutes, until the mixture has thickened.
4. At this point, remove from the heat and spoon an equal portion into each of two small cereal bowls.
5. This is when you top with blueberries and serve immediately.

NOTE: Remember, organic oat flakes, which are naturally free of gluten, are available at health food stores or better still online.

I suggest you look for brands that have not been packaged in a facility that also processes wheat.

Avocado Toast

Serves 1
Preparation Time: About 25 minutes
Tip:
This recipe is simple, delicious and a great way to start the day.
Ingredients:
1 teaspoon of organic distilled white vinegar
1 teaspoon of chopped organic cilantro
Fine sea salt (to taste)
Organic cilantro, organic mint leaf, or lime wedge for garnish (it is optional)
1 large egg from a pasture-raised chicken, at room temperature
1 small ripe organic avocado
Juice of ½ organic lime
1 slice of toasted Stone Age Bread
Organic crushed red pepper flakes (to taste)

Ingredients:

BRAIN WASH RECIPES

1. First, pour about 3 inches of cold water into a small deep saucepan.
2. After which you place over high heat and bring to a gentle simmer—you should see bubbles forming around the edge of the pan.
3. After that, add the vinegar.
4. Then, break the egg into a small fine-mesh sieve placed over a small bowl, allowing the albumen to drip into the bowl.
5. At this point, transfer the egg to a small custard-style cup. NOTE: this helps keep strands of egg white from forming in the water, resulting in a perfect round egg.
6. Furthermore, stir the simmering water with the handle of a wooden spoon to make a slight vortex.
7. After which you gently slide the egg into the center of the vortex.
8. This is when you simmer for about 2½ minutes, or until the egg white is firm and the yolk has just barely set.

9. In addition, using a slotted spoon or spatula, carefully transfer the egg to a clean warm custard-style cup.
10. After that, split the avocado in half lengthwise and, using a teaspoon, scoop out the flesh, discarding the pit.
11. Then place the flesh in a small shallow bowl and add the cilantro and lime juice.
12. At this point, season with sea salt and, using a kitchen fork, lightly mash.
13. This is when you spoon the avocado onto the toast, smoothing the top slightly; place the toast on a small plate.
14. Next, gently tip the egg from the warm cup into a slotted spoon. **NOTE:** if the egg has strands of egg white dripping off the edges, I suggest you carefully snip them off using kitchen shears.
15. You should slide the egg on top of the avocado toast.
16. Finally, sprinkle a bit of crushed red pepper flakes over the top and garnish with a sprig

of cilantro, a fresh mint leaf, or a wedge of lime if desired.

Breakfast Crepes

Makes about thirty 10-inch crepes
Preparation Time: About 15 minutes
Tips:

1. This recipe makes a wonderful breakfast dish. This breakfast of bread and dark chocolate is a traditional French a simple recipe, but you could also fill the crepes with scrambled eggs, berries, or grilled vegetables.
2. In this recipe you will need two nonstick 10-inch crepe pans, or you can cut the recipe in half and work with only one pan.

Ingredients:

1½ cups of organic almond flour

2–2½ cups of organic unsweetened almond milk, at room temperature

1 cup of finely grated organic dark chocolate, at least 80% cacao

6 large organic eggs from pasture-raised chickens, at room temperature, (lightly beaten)

1 teaspoon of fine sea salt

3 tablespoons of melted organic unsalted butter from grass-fed cows, + more for coating the pans and serving

1 teaspoon of pure organic vanilla extract

Directions:

1. First, break the eggs into a medium mixing bowl.
2. After which you whisk in the flour and salt.
3. After that, begin adding the milk in a slow, steady steam, whisking constantly.
4. Then, when you've added about half the milk, the batter should loosen, at which point you can add all the remaining milk along with 3 tablespoons of melted butter and the vanilla. NOTE: at this point the batter should lightly coat the back of a wooden spoon and have the consistency of half-and-half.
5. Meanwhile, heat two nonstick crepe pans over medium heat.

6. Furthermore, lightly coat each one with melted butter.
7. Then, using a small ladle, pour just enough crepe batter into one pan to coat the entire bottom.
8. After which you take the pan off the heat and lift and swirl it until the batter has spread to evenly coat the bottom.
9. This is when you begin making another crepe in the other hot pan; cook for about 45–60 seconds, or until the bottom is golden brown.
10. As each crepe is cooked, I suggest you drizzle it with melted butter and dust with grated chocolate.
11. In addition, using a silicone spatula, gently fold the crepe in half, then fold the half into quarters.
12. After that, flip the folded crepe out onto a plate and serve as you repeat the above steps with the remaining batter.

Remember, if you want to make the crepes in advance, place a parchment-lined cookie sheet in a 200°F oven.

13. Then, as each crepe finishes cooking, transfer it to the cookie sheet to keep warm. **NOTE:** do not stack; keep in a single layer.

    (**NOTE:** when you make your first crepe, the batter might stick to the pan and tear when you attempt to turn it. Remember that this indicates that the pan has not been properly seasoned or that there is a bit of residue on it from past crepe making. Often, the first crepe (or even the 2nd one) will stick because the pan is not at the correct temperature, but all subsequent crepes should pop right out. In the other hand, if the crepe looks as though it is pulling inward quickly, this indicates that the pan is too hot; if it doesn't set up almost immediately, the pan is too cold)

14. Finally, all this sounds daunting, but it really does become easy once you get started.

Greens with Eggs

Serves 4
Preparation Time: About 35 minutes
Tips:

1. In this recipe you can use any greens you like.
2. For variety and a stronger flavor, I suggest you use dandelion and/or mustard greens or mix them in with the chard and kale.

Ingredients:

2 large organic leeks, white part only, trimmed, well washed, and thinly sliced crosswise

1 large bunch organic Swiss chard (trimmed and shredded)

1 teaspoon of minced organic garlic

4 large eggs from pasture-raised chickens (at room temperature)

1 teaspoon of chopped fresh organic tarragon

½ teaspoon of organic ground sumac

¼ cup of organic extra virgin olive oil (divided)

2 organic shallots (peeled and thinly sliced crosswise)

1 bunch of organic lacinato kale, trimmed of tough stalks and shredded

1 tablespoon of freshly squeezed organic lemon juice

Fine sea salt and freshly ground organic black pepper (to taste)

½ teaspoon of organic crushed red pepper flakes

Directions:

1. Meanwhile, heat the oven to 350°F.
2. After which you heat 1 tablespoon of the oil in a large ovenproof frying pan over medium heat.
3. After that, add the leeks and shallots and cook, stirring frequently, for about 12 minutes, or until soft and golden brown.
4. Then, add the kale, chard, and garlic and continue to cook, stirring, for 3 minutes, or until the greens have wilted.

5. At this point, stir in the lemon juice along with another 2 tablespoons of the olive oil.
6. This is when you continue to cook for a minute or so, stirring to blend completely.
7. Furthermore, smooth out the top of the greens, then make four indentations in the top, each large enough to hold an egg.
8. After which you carefully slip an egg into each indentation; season with salt and pepper and transfer the pan to the preheated oven.
9. Then, bake for about 15 minutes, or until the eggs are just set.
10. In addition, while the eggs are baking, place the remaining olive oil in a small saucepan; add the tarragon, crushed red pepper, and sumac and place over medium heat.
11. After that, season with salt and pepper and cook, stirring occasionally, for about 3 minutes, or until the oil is hot and fragrant.
12. At this point, remove the pan from the oven.
13. Finally, drizzle the seasoned oil over the top and serve directly from the pan while hot.

Cauliflower Pancakes

Serves 4
Preparation Time: About 25 minutes
Tips:

1. Although this recipe makes a terrific breakfast or better still brunch dish, they are also a wonderful side dish for grilled meats, poultry, and/or fish. Remember, that the turmeric adds great color as well as a slightly tannic yet sweet flavor.

Ingredients:

1 small organic white onion (peeled and grated)

½ teaspoon of organic ground turmeric

Fine sea salt and freshly ground organic black pepper (to taste)

1 cup of full-fat organic sour cream from grass-fed cows (it is optional)

1-pound of organic cauliflower florets, including stems

1 teaspoon of grated organic garlic

3 large eggs from pasture-raised chickens, at room temperature, lightly beaten
⅓ cup of organic ghee from grass-fed animals
½ cup of chopped organic scallion greens

Directions:

1. Meanwhile, heat the oven to 200°F.
2. After which you place a cookie sheet lined with parchment paper in the oven.
3. Then, using a handheld box grater, grate the cauliflower through the medium holes.
4. After that, transfer the grated cauliflower in a large mixing bowl.
5. At this point, add the garlic, onion, and turmeric and toss to blend.
6. Furthermore, add the eggs and season with sea salt and pepper, stirring to combine completely; set aside for 10 minutes to allow the flavors to blossom.
7. After that, heat the ghee in a large frying pan over medium heat.

8. This is when you spoon in enough of the cauliflower mixture to make a flat cake about 3 inches in diameter.
9. Make sure you continue making cakes without crowding the pan.
10. Then, using the back of a metal spatula, flatten the cakes slightly, but allow them to get no larger than 4 inches in diameter.
11. In addition, fry for about 5 minutes, or until the bottom is golden brown and the pancakes have firmed enough to turn easily.
12. After which you lower the heat if they are browning too quickly; using the spatula—a fish spatula is a great tool for this—carefully turn the pancakes and fry for an additional 4 minutes, or until cooked through and golden brown. NOTE: if you flip them too quickly, they will fall apart.
13. As each one is cooked, I suggest you place it on the cookie sheet in the oven and continue making cakes until all the batter has been used.

14. Finally, when ready to serve, place the pancakes on a platter, sprinkle with sea salt and scallion greens, and serve with sour cream on the side if desired.

DELECTABLE BRAIN WASH APPETIZERS, SOUPS, SALADS, AND SMALL PLATES

Cauliflower Hummus

Serves 4 to 6
Preparation Time: About 12 minutes
Tips:

1. This recipe is a wonderful dip for crudités but also makes a terrific sandwich on the Stone Age Bread.
2. Remember, if you roast the cauliflower, the hummus will have a rich depth of flavor.

Ingredients:

4 cloves of organic garlic, peeled, or more to taste
1 teaspoon of organic ground cumin
Fine sea salt (to taste)
1 large head organic cauliflower, cut into florets and steamed until crisp tender
¼ cup of organic tahini
Juice of 1 organic lemon, or better still more to taste

Organic extra virgin olive oil (to taste)

Directions:

1. First, combine the garlic, cauliflower, tahini, and cumin in the bowl of a food processor fitted with a metal blade.
2. After which you begin processing and, with the motor running, add the lemon juice a bit at a time until you get the amount of acidity that you like.
3. After that, add just enough extra virgin olive oil to smooth out the mixture and add a bit of fruitiness; season with salt to taste.
4. At this point, scrape into a nonreactive container, cover, and refrigerate for up to one week.
5. Finally, serve at room temperature with an assortment of raw vegetables.

VARIATION:

Remember, if you want to add an elegant touch, I suggest you sprinkle the top with fresh organic pomegranate seeds or with a mix of organic black and toasted white sesame seeds before serving.

Madras Pea Soup

Serves 6
Preparation Time: About 40 minutes
Tips:

1. In this dish, the heat of the chili pepper and the savory East Indian spices make a great counterpoint to the sweet peas, cool yogurt, and aromatic herbs.
2. I recommend you use frozen organic peas for their beautiful color and consistent sweetness—fresh peas can be a bit dicey when it comes to color and starchiness.
3. Feel free to serve hot or cold, this is a filling soup that can, in larger portions, be used as a lunch or light supper entrée.

Ingredients:
¾ cup of chopped organic white onion
1 teaspoon of minced organic garlic
½ teaspoon of organic ground coriander
2 cups of dried organic split peas

One organic serrano or jalapeño chili pepper (stemmed and chopped, or more to taste)

Fine sea salt (to taste)

½ teaspoon of organic garam masala

Freshly ground organic black pepper (to taste)

1 tablespoon of chopped organic cilantro

6–8 sprigs organic cilantro or mint (it is optional)

1 tablespoon of organic coconut oil

1 tablespoon of minced organic ginger

2 teaspoons of toasted organic cumin seeds, ground in a mortar and pestle

½ teaspoon of organic ground cinnamon

1 small organic carrot, peeled, trimmed, and chopped

3 cups of Vegetable Stock or better still organic canned vegetable broth

Juice of 1 organic lemon

½ cup of plain full-fat organic yogurt from grass-fed animals, plus more for garnish (it is optional)

1 cup of frozen organic baby peas, thawed, drained, and patted dry

1 tablespoon of chopped organic mint

Directions:

1. First, heat the oil in a large heavy-bottom saucepan over medium heat.
2. After which you add the ginger, onion, and garlic and fry, stirring frequently, for about 5 minutes, or until the onions begin to take on some color.
3. After which you stir in the cumin, coriander, and cinnamon and sauté for 1 minute.
4. After that, add the carrot, chili pepper, split peas, and stock along with 3 cups of water and bring to a boil; season with salt.
5. At this point, lower the heat to a simmer and simmer for about 30 minutes, or until the peas are soft. NOTE: If the mixture gets too thick, I suggest you add stock or water ½ cup at a time.
6. This is when you remove from the heat and stir in the lemon juice, garam masala, and ½ cup yogurt.
7. Furthermore, pour into a blender—in batches, if necessary—and process to a smooth puree.

8. After that, pour the puree into a clean saucepan.
9. Then you place over medium heat and bring to a simmer, stirring frequently. (NOTE: do not allow the soup to boil, or the yogurt might curdle).
10. In addition, add the pepper, taste, and adjust the seasoning if necessary.
11. After which you stir in the peas, chopped cilantro, and chopped mint.
12. Finally, pour into shallow soup bowls and, if desired, garnish the center with a dollop of yogurt and a cilantro or mint sprig.

NOTE:

1. Remember, do not allow the frozen peas to sit at room temperature for too long, or they will shrivel.
2. I will suggest you remove them from the freezer just a bit before needed, transfer to a

strainer, and quickly defrost them under hot running water.

3. At this point, the hot water thaws and warms them rapidly so that they can be patted dry and added to the soup without chilling it down.

VARIATION:

1. Remember that this soup may also be served cold, after pureeing, cover and refrigerate for about 4 hours, or until well chilled.
2. Then, stir in the peas, cilantro, and mint just before serving and, if desired, garnish as above. (NOTE: the soup may also be frozen).

Garlic Soup

Serves 4 to 6
Preparation Time: About 40 minutes
Tip:
This recipe is a warming fall or winter filling-enough-to-be-a-main-course dish (NOTE: when you add cheese and some of our Stone Age Bread), and the aroma coming from the kitchen will make you ravenous.

Ingredients:

1 medium organic sweet onion, such as Vidalia (peeled and chopped)

2 organic whole cloves

2 sprigs of organic thyme

3 large organic egg yolks from pasture-raised chickens (at room temperature)

Freshly ground organic black pepper to taste (it is optional)

Freshly grated organic Parmesan cheese (for serving)

3 medium heads very fresh organic garlic (unpeeled)

2 organic bay leaves

2 organic sage leaves

Fine sea salt (to taste)

¼ cup of organic extra virgin olive oil

1 teaspoon of chopped organic flat-leaf parsley

1 teaspoon of chopped organic chives

Directions:

1. First, pour 2 quarts of water into a large saucepan and bring to a boil over high heat.
2. Then, while the water is coming to a boil, using your fingers, push all the dry, loose skin from the garlic heads.
3. After which you coarsely chop the heads, skin and all.
4. Furthermore, to the boiling water, add the chopped garlic along with the bay leaves, onion, cloves, sage leaves, and thyme sprigs.

5. After that, add salt to taste and return to a low simmer; simmer for about 25 minutes, or until the garlic is mushy.
6. In addition, while the broth is simmering, prepare the thickener.
7. After which you place the egg yolks in a small mixing bowl.
8. Then, using a whisk, beat the yolks until they are very light and quite thick. At this point, whisking constantly, add the oil in a slow, steady stream, beating until the mixture reaches the consistency of mayonnaise; cover and set aside until ready to use.
9. At this junction, when the garlic is mushy, remove the broth from the heat and strain through a fine-mesh sieve, discarding the solids; season the broth with salt and pepper.
10. This is when, you return the strained liquid to the saucepan and bring to a boil over medium heat.
11. In the meantime, scrape the thickener into a soup tureen or large serving bowl; once the

broth has come to a boil, remove it from the heat and, whisking the thickener constantly, slowly pour about a cup of the hot broth into the thickener; then pour in the remaining broth.

12. Finally, sprinkle chopped parsley and chives over the top.

13. You can serve individual portions with a healthy dose of grated Parmesan over the top.

Chicken Caesar Salad

Serves 4
Preparation Time: About 35 minutes
Tips:

1. This recipe contains what looks like a lot of ingredients, but they're not difficult to pull together.
2. However, the dressing and the chicken of this recipe can be made early in the day and the kale roasted an hour or so ahead of serving; then it's 1-2-3 to put it all together for this elegant version of a Caesar salad recipe.

Ingredients:

1 tablespoon of organic whole-grain mustard

1 teaspoon of organic anchovy paste

1 tablespoon of organic cider vinegar

Fine sea salt and freshly ground organic black pepper (to taste)

⅓ cup of finely grated organic Parmesan cheese

2 heads organic baby romaine lettuce (well washed and separated into leaves)

1 cup of shredded organic brussels sprouts

½ cup of sliced raw unsalted organic almonds (toasted)

3 large organic egg yolks from pasture-raised chickens (at room temperature)

1 teaspoon of organic Dijon mustard

1 teaspoon of Roasted Garlic (here)

½ cup of organic extra virgin olive oil, divided

4 boneless, skinless organic chicken breasts from pasture-raised chickens (about 6 ounces each)

8 organic kale leaves (trimmed of their tough stalks)

3 cups of organic baby spinach leaves

½ cup of thinly sliced organic radishes

Directions:

1. First, combine the mustards, garlic, egg yolks, anchovy paste, and vinegar in a small mixing bowl.
2. After which you slowly pour in ¼ cup of the olive oil, whisking to emulsify.

3. After that, season with salt and pepper and set aside.
4. Meanwhile, heat the oven to 300°F.
5. Then, line a baking sheet with parchment paper and set aside.
6. In the meantime, heat an outdoor grill or preheat a stovetop grill pan over high heat.
7. After which you trim the chicken of any membrane or sinew; generously rub all sides with about 2 tablespoons of the remaining olive oil and season with salt and pepper.
8. Then, place the chicken breasts on the hot grill or pan and cook, turning frequently, for about 10 minutes, or until just cooked through and the temperature on an instant-read thermometer reaches 155°F.
9. At this point, remove from the heat and set aside. NOTE: The chicken will continue to cook as it rests and should reach at least 160°F.
10. Furthermore, while the chicken is cooking, prepare the kale; combine the remaining olive oil with the Parmesan cheese and salt

and pepper to taste in a small bowl, whisking to blend completely.

11. Then, using a pastry brush, coat both sides of the kale leaves with the mixture.

12. After that, place the seasoned kale leaves on the prepared baking sheet in the preheated oven and roast for about 20 minutes, or until the kale is lightly browned and crisp.

13. This is when you remove from the oven and set aside; when ready to serve, cut the chicken crosswise into thin slices and set aside.

14. In addition, combine the radishes, romaine, brussels sprouts, spinach, and almonds in a large mixing bowl.

15. After which you add the sliced chicken along with about half the mustard dressing and toss to combine.

16. Then place equal portions of the salad on each of four luncheon plates; place an equal portion of roasted kale on top of each serving.

17. Finally, serve immediately with the remaining dressing on the side.

Chicory Salad with Tahini Dressing

Serves 4
Preparation Time: About 15 minutes
Tips:
Try to find some purple, some green, and some speckled chicories when choosing your greens to make the salad visually exciting, too.

Ingredients:

½ cup of coarsely chopped unsalted organic walnuts (toasted)

About ¼ cup organic pomegranate seeds (it is optional)

¾ pound mixed organic chicories, such as frisée, radicchio, Belgian endive, or other bitter leafy greens

Tahini Dressing to taste (stated below)

Directions:

1. First, combine the greens and walnuts in a large salad bowl.

2. After which you add just enough dressing to lightly coat and toss to blend well.
3. Then, serve immediately with pomegranate seeds strewn over the top, if desired.

Directions for the Tahini Dressing:

Makes about 6 tablespoons
Preparation Time: About 15 minutes
Ingredients:
½ teaspoon of minced organic garlic
Fine sea salt and freshly ground organic black pepper (to taste)
2 tablespoons of organic tahini
Zest and juice of ½ small organic orange
3 tablespoons of organic extra virgin olive oil
Directions:

1. First, combine the tahini with the garlic and orange zest and juice in a small mixing bowl.
2. After which you slowly whisk in the olive oil and season with salt and pepper.

3. Remember, if the dressing seems too thick or grainy, I suggest you add cool water a tablespoon at a time until the desired consistency is reached. (NOTE: the dressing should resemble thick cream).

Sesame Beef Kebabs with Avocado Dipping Sauce

Makes 28 pieces
Preparation Time: About 15 minutes, plus one hour for soaking skewers
Tips:

1. This recipe would be a fun appetizer or snack for a summer grilling party; you could get everything together and then let your guests grill their own kebabs.
2. However, the dipping sauce adds a bit of zest, but the kebabs are great on their own, too.

Ingredients:

Fine sea salt and freshly cracked organic black pepper (to taste)

1 recipe Avocado Dipping Sauce (below; it is optional)

2 organic New York strip or better still rib-eye steaks from grass-fed cows, about 1 pound each, trimmed of all fat

1 cup of organic sesame seeds

1 cup of organic avocado oil

Directions:

1. First, place twenty-eight 8-inch bamboo skewers in cold water and let soak for at least 1 hour.
2. After which you drain well, but do not allow the skewers to dry out.
3. Then, using a sharp knife, trim a thin edge off the sides of each steak to make two neat rectangles, each about 7 inches long by 4 inches wide by 1 inch thick.
4. After that, cut each steak crosswise into 7 pieces, each about 4 inches long and 1 inch wide.
5. At this point, place the 14 pieces of meat alongside one another with the length facing away from you.
6. This is when you weave two bamboo skewers up through each piece of meat so that when the strip is cut in half down the middle after cooking you will have two skewers of beef of

equal size. (NOTE: The skewers may be assembled up to this point and stored, covered, and refrigerated, for up to 24 hours or frozen for up to three months.)

7. Furthermore, when ready to cook, place the sesame seeds on a clean flat surface.
8. After that, season the meat with salt and pepper, then roll each skewer in sesame seeds to completely cover.
9. Then, pour the oil into a nonstick griddle or stovetop grill pan set over medium-high heat.
10. At this point when the oil is shimmering, place the skewers in the hot oil and sear, turning occasionally, for about 2 minutes, or until the meat is nicely browned but still rare in the center.
11. This is when you transfer the skewers to a cutting board and cut each one in half to make two smaller skewers of equal size.
12. In addition, lay the skewers out on a serving platter cut side up to show the rareness of the meat.

BRAIN WASH RECIPES

13. Finally, serve immediately with the dipping sauce on the side if desired.

Avocado Dipping Sauce

Makes about 1 cup
Preparation Time: About 15 minutes
Ingredients:
⅓ cup of plain full-fat organic yogurt from grass-fed animals

1 teaspoon of grated organic ginger

Freshly grated organic green chili pepper to taste (it is optional)

1 large ripe organic avocado (peeled and pitted)

2 tablespoons of grated organic red onion

Fine sea salt and freshly ground organic black pepper (to taste)

Directions:

1. First, place the yogurt, avocado, onion, and ginger in the bowl of a food processor fitted with a metal blade.
2. After which you process until very smooth.
3. Then, you taste and season with salt and pepper and, if desired, freshly grated chili pepper.

Grilled Clams with Citrus-Herb Sauce

Serves 4 to 6
Preparation Time: About 15 minutes
Tips:

1. This recipe is a perfect summer appetizer, cocktail tidbit, or snack and its grilling clams is quick and easy to do while chatting with guests.
2. Remember, when the clams are topped with a light, refreshing herb sauce, there is nothing more elegant or good for you. (NOTE: The sauce is also terrific on poultry, grilled fish, or meat).

Ingredients:

Citrus-Herb Sauce to taste (check below)
3 dozen wild clams, well-scrubbed (check the Note)

Directions:

1. Meanwhile, heat an outdoor grill to high.
2. After which you place the clams on the grill with the flatter side up. (**NOTE:** this will help hold the juices in the rounder side as the clams open from the heat).
3. After that, grill for about 4 minutes, or until the clams open.
4. Then, as they open, remove the clams from the grill, dollop with a bit of the sauce, and eat them hot, straight from the shell.
5. **Remember,** fresh wild clams need to be soaked in salt water, better still the same water they came from, to allow them to expunge the sand from their shells.

Citrus-Herb Sauce

Makes about 2 cups

Ingredients:

½ cup of chopped organic leeks, including some green parts

2 tablespoons of chopped organic oregano

½ teaspoon of freshly grated organic orange zest

1 cup of organic extra virgin olive oil

Fine sea salt (to taste)

2 cups of chopped organic flat-leaf parsley

¼ cup of chopped organic cilantro

1 tablespoon of chopped organic garlic

Juice and zest of 1 organic lemon

¼ cup of organic champagne vinegar

Directions:

1. First, combine the leeks, cilantro, parsley, garlic, oregano, and orange zest in the bowl of a food processor fitted with a metal blade and pulse until just minced.
2. After which you add the lemon juice and zest and process to just incorporate.

3. After that, scrape the mixture into a nonreactive container.
4. Then stir in the oil and vinegar.
5. Finally, season with salt, cover, and refrigerate until ready to use.

DELECTABLE BRAIN WASH ENTRÉES

Lamb with Mustard Sauce

Serves 4
Preparation Time: About 30 minutes
Tips:
This recipe is easy to double or triple the spices to coat as many lamb racks as you need.

Ingredients:

1¼ teaspoons of organic ground turmeric

½ teaspoon of organic chili powder

1 (about 8-rib) rack of organic grass-fed lamb, about 1½ pounds

3 tablespoons of organic whole-grain mustard

1 teaspoon of organic garam masala

2 tablespoons of organic coconut oil

Fine sea salt (to taste)

Directions:

1. Meanwhile, heat the oven to 425°F.
2. After which you combine the mustard, garam masala, turmeric, chili powder, and

coconut oil in a small bowl, stirring to blend completely.
3. After that, season with salt; generously rub the mustard mixture over the lamb.
4. Then, place the coated meat in a roasting pan and roast for about 20 minutes, or until an instant-read thermometer inserted into the thickest part reads 140°F (NOTE: which will yield rare meat if served immediately).
5. At this point, place the rack on a cutting board and let rest for about 10 minutes, or until the thermometer registers 150°F for medium rare.
6. Finally, using a chef's knife, cut through each rack along the bone and serve 2 chops per person.

Deviled Cornish Game Hens

Serves 4 to 6
Time required: About 25 minutes
Tips:

1. This recipe could easily be prepared with chicken, pork, turkey, or seafood.
2. Remember, that the sauce would also be very tasty served with cauliflower steaks or grilled vegetables.

Ingredients:

2 fresh organic red or better still green hot chili peppers, stemmed and seeded, or more to taste

¼ cup of minced organic yellow onion

Fine sea salt (to taste)

Juice of 1 organic lemon

1 tablespoon of organic tamarind paste dissolved in 2 tablespoons warm water

1 cup of unsweetened organic coconut milk

1 tablespoon of minced organic garlic

3 whole organic pasture-raised Cornish game hens, cleaned and split in half lengthwise

Directions:

1. Meanwhile, heat an outdoor grill to high.
2. After which you strain the tamarind through a fine-mesh sieve, pressing on the solids to extract all the liquid. (**NOTE:** you should have around 1 tablespoon).
3. After that, discard the solids; in the bowl of a food processor, combine the tamarind liquid with the coconut milk, chili peppers, onion, and garlic and process until smooth.
4. Then, season with salt to taste.
5. At this point, generously rub the hens with lemon juice; place on the preheated grill and grill each side for 2 minutes.
6. This is when you remove from the grill and set aside. (NOTE: Keep the grill hot).
7. Furthermore, using the flat side of a cleaver or a heavy-bottom frying pan, pound each hen half to flatten it slightly.
8. After that, place the flattened hens, skin side down, in a large frying pan.

9. Then, add the tamarind mixture and place over medium heat.
10. This is when you bring to a boil, then lower the heat and simmer for 6 minutes.
11. In addition, immediately remove the hens from the sauce and return to the hot grill.
12. After which you grill, skin side down, for 4 minutes, or until crisp.
13. Finally, remove from the grill and serve immediately with or without the sauce from the pan.

Almost Tandoori Chicken

Serves 4 to 6

Preparation Time: About 1 hour, plus 24 hours for marinating

Tips:

This recipe may not look quite as glorious as a tandoor-burnished traditional Indian chicken, but it is still very tasty. However, just a hint of spice permeates the extremely tender, moist meat.

Ingredients:

2 tablespoons of freshly squeezed organic lime juice

¾ cup of chopped organic yellow onion

1 teaspoon of minced fresh organic garlic

2 teaspoons of organic garam masala

1 whole organic pasture-raised roasting chicken (about 3½–4 pounds)

2½ cups of plain full-fat organic yogurt from grass-fed animals

½–1 organic hot red chili pepper (seeded and chopped)

1 tablespoon of minced fresh organic ginger

1 tablespoon of organic paprika

1 teaspoon of organic ground turmeric

Directions:

1. First, combine the yogurt and lime juice in the bowl of a food processor fitted with a metal blade and process to just combine.
2. After which you add the onion, chili pepper, ginger, and garlic and process to blend.
3. After that, add the paprika, garam masala, and turmeric and process until almost smooth.
4. At this point, cut small slits in the skin of the chicken so it will absorb the marinade, then place it in a large resealable plastic bag.
5. This is when you add the yogurt mixture, seal, and toss to cover well.
6. Furthermore, place in the refrigerator and allow to marinate for 24 hours (but no longer), turning the bag from time to time to

ensure that the entire chicken is tenderized by the marinade.

7. Then, about 30 minutes before you are ready to roast, preheat your oven to 500°F or make a very hot charcoal fire on one side of an outdoor grill—you will want the temperature to reach 500°F before you cook the chicken.
8. After that, remove the chicken from the plastic bag and turn it so that excess marinade drips out of the cavity; discard the marinade.
9. At this point, place the chicken on a rack in a roasting pan or on the grill rack on the far opposite side of the fire.
10. After which you cover and begin roasting, turning the chicken occasionally to ensure that it is cooking evenly.
11. In addition, add charcoal as necessary to the grill to maintain the hot fire. NOTE: In the oven, this should take no more than 40 minutes; on the grill, it can take about 2 hours for the chicken to be perfectly cooked throughout.

BRAIN WASH RECIPES

12. Finally, remove from the oven or grill and let rest for about 15 minutes before cutting into pieces.

Whole Roasted Striped Bass

Serves 6
Preparation Time: About 40 minutes
Tips:
Remember, that you can adapt this recipe to any whole firm fish, or, if you prefer, you can use nice thick fillets of any sweet, firm-fleshed wild fish, such as salmon or halibut.

Ingredients:

2 unpeeled organic lemons (well washed and thinly sliced crosswise)

10 sprigs organic flat-leaf parsley, (+ more for garnish if desired)

2 tablespoons of freshly squeezed organic lemon juice

2 large organic fennel bulbs (thinly sliced crosswise)

½ cup of organic dry white wine

2 whole wild striped bass, 3 pounds each (gutted and cleaned)

10 sprigs of organic tarragon, + more for garnish if desired

3 tablespoons of organic extra virgin olive oil

Fine sea salt and freshly ground organic black pepper (to taste)

3 cups (about 2 pounds) peeled and sliced organic shallots (blanched)

Directions:

1. Meanwhile, heat the oven to 450°F.
2. After which you rinse the fish and pat dry, both inside and out.
3. After that, layer half the lemon slices in the cavity of one of the fish.
4. Then, place about 5 sprigs each of tarragon and parsley on top of the lemons. Make sure you repeat with the other fish.
5. At this point, combine the olive oil and lemon juice in a small bowl.
6. Furthermore, using your hands, generously coat both fish with the oil mixture.

7. After that, season both sides with salt and pepper.
8. Then, combine the fennel and shallots in a shallow roasting pan large enough to hold both fish.
9. This is when you season with salt and pepper and smooth the vegetables out to an even layer.
10. In addition, pour the wine into the pan, then place the fish on top of the vegetables.
11. After which you place the pan in the preheated oven and roast, turning the vegetables occasionally, for about 25 minutes, or until the vegetables are tender and an instant-read thermometer inserted into the thickest part of the fish reads 135°F.
12. Then, remove the pan from the oven and allow the fish to rest for 5 minutes.
13. However, using two spatulas, carefully lift each fish from the roasting pan onto a serving platter.
14. Finally, spoon the fennel-shallot mixture around each fish and, if desired, garnish

with chopped tarragon or parsley and fresh lemon slices.

Salmon with Green Sauce

Serves 4

Preparation Time: About 15 minutes

Tips:

1. Remember, this is such an easy recipe that you can pull it together in a few minutes.
2. This recipe is perfect for a weekday meal or even a celebratory dinner, because it looks so pretty on the plate.

Ingredients:

⅓ cup of organic unsalted butter from grass-fed cows

1 tablespoon of organic coconut oil

Organic ground cumin for dusting

2 bunches of organic arugula (or better still spinach or any other bitter green), well washed

Fine sea salt and freshly ground organic black pepper (to taste)

4 skinless wild salmon fillets (6 ounces each)

Directions:

1. First, place the arugula in boiling water for about 30 seconds to blanch.
2. After which you drain well and pat dry.
3. After that, transfer the blanched greens to a blender (or better still food processor fitted with a metal blade) and process to a sauce like consistency, adding a bit of warm water as needed to smooth out.
4. At this point, scrape the puree into a small saucepan, add the butter, salt, and pepper, and set over low heat to warm through.
5. This is when you remove from the heat and keep warm. (Note: The puree can be made in advance and reheated in a double boiler.)
6. Furthermore, heat the coconut oil in a large frying pan over high heat.
7. After that, season the salmon with salt and pepper and dust both sides with cumin.
8. In addition, place in the hot pan and sear, turning once, for about 6 minutes, or until nicely colored on the exterior and rare in the center.

9. Finally, place a salmon fillet in the center of each of four serving plates and drizzle the green puree around the edge; serve immediately.

Whole Roasted Salmon with Sunchokes and Leeks

Serves 6

Preparation Time: About 30 minutes

Tip:

Remember, if you can't get a whole six-pound salmon for this recipe, don't hesitate to use a smaller fish or just roast one side of a larger salmon.

However, this recipe is a lovely dish for guests, filling them with the prebiotic
goodness of the sunchokes and leeks; can be prepared with striped bass or any other slightly fatty fish and served hot or at room temperature.

Ingredients:

3 branches of organic rosemary, 5 inches each, or other herb of choice

1 whole wild salmon, about 6 pounds, gutted and cleaned, head and tail left on, rinsed and patted dry

1 tablespoon of organic coconut oil

1 teaspoon of fresh organic rosemary leaves

Organic watercress sprigs for garnish (it is optional)

1½ pounds of small organic sun chokes (scrubbed)

1 unpeeled organic lemon (sliced crosswise)

Fine sea salt and freshly ground organic black pepper (to taste)

6 organic leeks, including a trace of the green parts, trimmed, well washed, and sliced lengthwise

Organic lemon wedges for garnish (it is optional)

Directions:

1. First, bring a large pot of salted water to a boil over high heat.
2. After which you add the sun chokes, lower the heat, and simmer for about 5 minutes, or until just slightly cooked.
3. After that, drain and pat dry; set aside.
4. Meanwhile, heat the oven to 375°F.

5. At this point, place the rosemary branches and lemon slices in the cavity of the fish; season with salt and pepper.
6. Then, using a pastry brush, lightly coat the top of the salmon with coconut oil.
7. Furthermore, place the reserved sun chokes and the leeks in a roasting pan large enough to hold the salmon.
8. After which you sprinkle the vegetables with the rosemary leaves and season with salt and pepper.
9. This is when you lay the salmon on top of the vegetables; place in the preheated oven and roast for about 15 minutes per inch of thickness of the fish, or until an instant-read thermometer reads 135°F when inserted into the thickest part of the salmon.
10. In addition, remove the pan from the oven and allow the fish to rest for 10 minutes.
11. Finally, serve the salmon and vegetables garnished with lemon wedges and watercress, if desired.

Vegetable Lasagna

Serves 4 to 8
Preparation Time: About 1½ hours
Tips:

1. This recipe is a rich meal, and the pasta and meat won't be missed at all; it's also a great dish to carry to parties, potlucks, or almost any gathering.
2. However, guests will be grateful for the introduction of this lighter, more healthful version of the beloved Italian classic recipe.

Ingredients:
Fine sea salt (to taste)
1 cup of finely diced organic yellow onion
1 can (about 28 ounces) plus 1 cup organic crushed tomatoes
2 teaspoons of organic dried oregano
Freshly ground organic black pepper (to taste)
2 cups of Ricotta Cheese (here)

1 large organic egg from pasture-raised chickens (at room temperature)

3½ pounds of organic zucchini

2 tablespoons of organic extra virgin olive oil

1 tablespoon of smashed organic garlic

1 tablespoon of organic dried basil

¼ teaspoon of organic crushed red pepper flakes

5½ cups of shredded organic full-fat mozzarella cheese from grass-fed animals (divided)

2 cups of grated organic Parmesan cheese (divided)

Directions:

1. Meanwhile, heat the oven to 375°F.
2. After which you line two baking sheets with parchment paper; set aside.
3. Then, using a handheld vegetable slicer or a mandolin, cut the zucchini lengthwise into ¼-inch-thick slices.
4. After that, lay the slices in a single layer on the prepared baking sheets.
5. At this point, sprinkle the slices with salt and set aside for 10 minutes. (NOTE: This will

draw some of the moisture out of the vegetables and prevent the lasagna from becoming runny).

6. Furthermore, after 10 minutes, use a paper towel to gently pat the zucchini dry.
7. After that, transfer the baking sheets to the preheated oven and roast for about 12 minutes, or until the zucchini slices are beginning to color around the edges; remove from the oven and set aside.
8. This is when you heat the olive oil in a large saucepan over medium heat.
9. In addition, add the onion and garlic and cook, stirring frequently, for about 4 minutes, or just until the vegetables are starting to soften.
10. After which you add the tomatoes along with the basil, oregano, and red pepper flakes; season with salt and pepper and bring to a simmer.
11. At this point, cook, stirring occasionally, for about 15 minutes, or until the sauce has thickened slightly.

12. Remember to taste and, if necessary, season with additional salt and pepper.
13. This is when you combine 2 cups of the mozzarella with the Ricotta Cheese and 1 cup of the Parmesan in the bowl of a food processor fitted with a metal blade.
14. Then, add the egg and season with salt and pepper; pulse until the mixture is completely smooth.
15. However, spoon about 1 cup of the tomato mixture on the bottom of a 12 × 16-inch baking pan; lay about one-fourth of the zucchini slices on top, followed by about 1 cup of the cheese mixture, taking care that it covers the zucchini completely.
16. Feel free to top with a layer of about 1 cup mozzarella and about ¼ cup Parmesan; repeat the layering two more times.
17. You can now add a layer of zucchini slices followed by the remaining ½ cup of mozzarella.
18. Finish with the remaining ¼ cup of Parmesan; place the lasagna in the

preheated oven and bake for 30 minutes. NOTE: increase the oven temperature to 500°F and continue to bake for 5 minutes, or until the cheese is golden brown and the lasagna is very hot and bubbling.
19. Finally, remove from the oven and set on a wire rack to settle for about 15 minutes before cutting and serving.

Grilled Cauliflower and Broccoli Steaks with Eggplant

Serves 4
Time required: About 45 minutes
Tips:
Remember, if you don't have time to make the eggplant or the dressing, I suggest you grill the "steaks" and drizzle with a vinaigrette or some extra virgin olive oil and balsamic vinegar.

Ingredients:

¾ cup of organic extra virgin olive oil, + more for coating grill pan

Organic cayenne pepper (to taste)

1 large head organic broccoli (trimmed and cut into 4 equal pieces)

1 tablespoon of mashed Roasted Garlic (check Note)

Organic cracked black pepper (to taste)

Organic ground sumac for garnish (it is optional)

1 organic globe eggplant (about 2 pounds), trimmed

Fine sea salt (to taste)

1 large head organic cauliflower (trimmed and cut lengthwise into 1-inch-thick slices)

¼ cup of organic oregano leaves

1 tablespoon of organic fennel seeds

Tahini Dressing to taste

Directions:

1. Meanwhile, heat an outdoor grill or a stovetop grill pan over high heat.
2. After which you line two large baking pans with parchment; set aside.
3. After that, cut the eggplant in half lengthwise and, using about ¼ cup of the olive oil, generously oil each half.
4. Then, place the eggplant cut side down on the grill or grill pan.
5. At this point, grill, turning occasionally, for about 30 minutes, or until the flesh is crinkled and golden brown and the skin has blackened and charred.
6. This is when you remove the eggplant from the heat and slip the skin off the flesh.

7. Furthermore, season with the salt and cayenne pepper and stir, adding just enough olive oil to create a soft, smooth puree; set aside but keep warm.
8. Then, while the eggplant is cooking, prepare the cauliflower and broccoli.
9. Pour the remaining olive oil in a small bowl; add the oregano, Roasted Garlic, and fennel seeds.
10. After that, season with salt and cracked pepper; using a pastry brush, generously coat both sides of the cauliflower and broccoli with the seasoned oil.
11. At this point you place the vegetables on the lined baking sheets to marinate for a few minutes.

NOTE: when the eggplant comes off the grill, I suggest you carefully transfer the vegetable steaks to the grill.

12. In addition, grill, turning once, for about 6 minutes, or until the steaks are just barely tender.
13. After which you spoon an equal portion of the eggplant into the center of each of four dinner plates; layer a cauliflower steak onto the eggplant and place a broccoli steak at its side.
14. Finally, drizzle with Tahini Dressing and garnish with a sprinkle of ground sumac if desired.
15. Make sure you serve immediately.

NOTE: if you want to make Roasted Garlic, first, preheat the oven to 350 F. After which you lightly coat either unpeeled whole heads of organic garlic or peeled individual cloves with organic extra virgin olive oil, wrap in aluminum foil, and place on a baking pan in the preheated oven. **NOTE:** If you're serving whole heads on a platter with grilled meats, make a nice, neat slice off the top before roasting. Remember, whole heads will take about

25

minutes to become soft and aromatic; individual cloves will take about 12 minutes.

Directions on how to make roasted garlic puree:

1. First, roast whole heads as directed above and, when they're soft and
2. aromatic, cut off the tops and squeeze out the lush, soft flesh.

Remember one large head will usually yield about 2 tablespoons of puree.

3. Furthermore, roasted garlic is rich, deeply flavorful, and not at all pungent.

DELECTABLE BRAIN WASH SIDES

Jicama Slaw

Serves 4 to 6

Time required: About 20 minutes

Tips:

1. This side dish goes splendidly with grilled wild fish, chicken, or pork, particularly **NOTE:** if it has a little spice added.
2. This recipe is a refreshing and healthful substitute for regular coleslaw and would be most welcome at a summertime barbecue or picnic.

Ingredients:

2 cloves of organic garlic (peeled)

¼ cup of organic extra virgin olive oil

1 organic red onion (peeled and cut into julienne strips)

1 bunch of organic scallions (thinly sliced diagonally)

Juice of two small organic oranges

Juice of one organic lime

1 bunch of organic cilantro leaves

3 small organic jicamas (peeled and cut into julienne strips)

1 bunch of organic mint leaves (cut into slivers)

Directions:

1. First, combine the citrus juices, cilantro, garlic, and olive oil in a blender and process until almost smooth; set aside until ready to use.
2. After which you place the jicama, mint, onions, and scallions in a large salad bowl.
3. Then, add enough of the dressing to lightly coat the salad.
4. Finally, serve immediately.

Sautéed Asparagus

Serves 4 to 6
Time required: About 10 minutes
Tip:
Remember, this piquant mixture works well as an accompaniment to almost any meat, poultry, or game and as a luncheon course topped with poached or scrambled eggs.

Ingredients:

2 small organic shallots (peeled and thinly sliced)

2 sprigs of organic thyme leaves

½ tablespoon of organic sherry vinegar

2 tablespoons of organic ghee from grass-fed animals

2 bunches of organic green asparagus (trimmed and cut in half)

1 pickled chili pepper (seeded and minced)

Fine sea salt and freshly ground organic white pepper to taste

Directions:

1. First, heat the ghee in a large sauté pan over medium heat.

2. After which you add the shallots and cook, stirring frequently, for 3 minutes, or until translucent.
3. After that, add the asparagus, thyme, and chili pepper.
4. At this point, season with salt and pepper and cook, tossing and stirring frequently, for about 7 minutes, or until the asparagus is just crisp-tender.
5. Then, about a minute before the asparagus is ready, deglaze the pan with the sherry vinegar.
6. Finally, toss and remove from the heat.
7. Make sure you serve immediately.

Zucchini and Parsnip Noodles with Celery Root in Broccoli Sauce

Serves 4
Time required: About 20 minutes
Tips:
This recipe makes a delicious side dish or even a main course.
Ingredients:
½ cup of finely grated organic Parmesan cheese, + more for sprinkling

Fine sea salt (to taste)

2 cloves organic garlic (peeled and thinly sliced)

1 tablespoon of freshly grated organic lemon zest

½ pound of organic celery root (shredded)

8 cups (approx. 1 pound) organic broccoli florets

⅓ cup of unsalted raw organic cashews

¼ cup of organic extra virgin olive oil, + more for drizzling

One organic hot red chili pepper, trimmed, seeded, and finely chopped, or more to taste

1½ pounds of organic zucchini noodles

½ pound of organic parsnip noodles

Directions:

1. First, combine the broccoli, cashews, ½ cup Parmesan, and salt in the bowl of a food processor fitted with a metal blade.
2. After which you process until fine crumbs form.
3. After that, heat ¼ cup oil in a large frying pan over medium heat.
4. Then, add the garlic and chili pepper and sauté, stirring frequently, for about 2 minutes, or until the garlic is soft but not colored.
5. At this point, add the broccoli mixture along with the lemon zest and continue to cook, stirring, for about 10 minutes, or until the mixture is browning and very fragrant.
6. This is when you add the parsnip, zucchini, and celery root and cook, tossing, for about 3 minutes, or until the noodles are coated with the sauce and warmed through.

7. Finally, remove from the heat and serve drizzled with more olive oil and sprinkled with Parmesan cheese.

Sunchoke Gratin

Serves 4
Preparation Time: About 35 minutes
Tip:
In this recipe I added a healthy dose of black pepper to offset the sweetness and accent the mellowness of the finished dish and like many of the side dishes in this chapter, this gratin can also work as a main course for lunch or a light supper.

Ingredients:
1 tablespoon of organic avocado oil
1 pound of organic sunchokes, peeled and cut crosswise into ⅛-inch-thick slices
Fine sea salt and freshly ground organic black pepper (to taste)
2 ounces grated organic Cheddar cheese from grass-fed cows
2 tablespoons of organic unsalted butter from grass-fed cows
1 large organic white onion (peeled and cut lengthwise into thin wedges)

1 tablespoon of chopped organic thyme leaves

¼ cup of organic crème fraîche from grass-fed cows

Directions:

1. First, combine the butter and oil in a large ovenproof frying pan over medium heat.
2. After which you add the onion and cook, stirring frequently, for about 10 minutes, or until the onion is soft and beginning to color.
3. After that, add the sunchokes and thyme and generously season with salt and pepper.
4. Then, add ½ cup water and bring to a simmer.
5. At this point, lower the heat, cover, and cook for about 20 minutes, or until the sunchokes are very tender.
6. This is when you uncover and simmer until the pan juices are reduced to a thick glaze, adding water a tablespoon at a time if necessary.
7. Meanwhile, heat the broiler.

8. Furthermore, dollop the crème fraîche over the top of the sunchokes and spread it into an even layer.
9. After that, sprinkle the cheese over the top and immediately transfer to the broiler.
10. In addition, broil for about 4 minutes, or until the top is golden brown and the edges are bubbling.
11. Finally, remove from the broiler and serve.

Leeks and Swiss Chard with Coconut Milk

Serves 4
Preparation Time: About 20 minutes
Tip:
In this recipe you can use kale or another green in place of the chard, but try not to use a very bitter green because it will overpower the sweetness of the leeks.

Ingredients:

2 tablespoons of organic ghee from grass-fed cows

½ pound of organic Swiss chard leaves, trimmed of tough stalks and cut crosswise into ribbons

¼ teaspoon of organic ground turmeric

1⅔ cups of organic unsweetened coconut milk

5 organic leeks, including white and tender green parts (trimmed and well washed)

2 cloves of organic garlic (peeled and sliced)

1 teaspoon of organic hot curry powder

Fine sea salt (to taste)

¼ cup of chopped toasted organic unsalted nuts, such as a mix of almonds, cashews, walnuts, and macadamia nuts

Directions:

1. First, cut the leeks crosswise into ½-inch-thick diagonal slices.
2. After which you heat the ghee in a large frying pan over medium-low heat. After that, add the garlic and fry, stirring frequently, for a couple of minutes, or just until it softens but hasn't taken on any color.
3. Then, add the leeks along with the chard and continue to cook, stirring frequently, for about 5 minutes, or until the vegetables begin to soften.
4. Furthermore, add the curry powder and turmeric and season with salt.
5. At this point, cook, stirring, for another 3 minutes, or until the leeks are tender.
6. This is when you add the coconut milk and bring to a simmer.

7. In addition, simmer for about 4 minutes, or just until the mixture
8. begins to bubble.
9. Finally, remove from the heat, scrape into a serving bowl, and sprinkle with chopped nuts.
10. Make sure you serve immediately.

Broccoli with Shallots and Red Pepper

Serves 4
Preparation Time: About 15 minutes
Tips:
Don't overcook the broccoli in this simple but tasty recipe, because you want it to be slightly crisp and not one bit wilted.

Remember, you can also add some crushed red pepper flakes if you are in the mood for some spice.

Ingredients:

2 tablespoons of organic coconut oil

1 small organic red bell pepper (trimmed, seeded, deveined, and finely diced)

Fine sea salt and freshly ground organic black pepper (to taste)

8 cups (about 1 pound) organic broccoli florets

2 organic shallots (peeled and cut crosswise into thin slices)

1 teaspoon of minced organic garlic

Directions:

1. First, place the broccoli in the basket of a steamer with an inch or so of water in the bottom.
2. Then, make sure the steamer basket does not touch the water.
3. After which you cover, place over high heat, and bring the water to a boil.
4. After that, steam the broccoli for 2 minutes, then immediately remove the steamer basket from the heat and set aside.
5. At this point, heat the oil in a large frying pan over medium heat.
6. This is when you add the shallots, bell pepper, and garlic and fry, stirring frequently, for about 5 minutes, or until the vegetables begin to soften.
7. Furthermore, add the steamed broccoli, season with salt and pepper, and cook, stirring, for another minute or two.

8. Finally, transfer to a serving bowl and serve immediately.

Dandelion Greens with Onions

Serves 4
Preparation Time: About 30 minutes
Tips:

1. Remember that dandelion greens are best in the spring, when they are small, young, tender, and not as bitter as the older greens will be.
2. However, they are an excellent source of vitamins and prebiotics and should be eaten far more often than they are.
3. Make sure you pick your own, but you must make sure they are pristine, without having come into contact with toxic sprays or animal contaminants.

Ingredients:
¼ cup + 1 tablespoon organic extra virgin olive oil
1 cup of chopped organic shallots
¾ cup of chopped mixed organic herbs, such as cilantro, parsley, chives, and basil
Juice of one organic lemon

2 pounds of organic dandelion greens, tough stems removed, chopped

1 large organic onion (peeled and cut crosswise into thin rings)

1 tablespoon of chopped organic garlic

Fine sea salt (to taste)

Directions:

1. First, bring a large pot of salted water to a boil over high heat.
2. After which you add the chopped dandelion greens and boil for about 3 minutes, or just until tender.
3. After that, drain the greens through a fine-mesh strainer, then transfer to a large clean kitchen towel.
4. At this point, twist the towel together and wring the greens as dry as you can; set aside.
5. Then, place ¼ cup of the oil in a large frying pan over medium-high heat.
6. Furthermore, when the oil is very hot but not shimmering, add the sliced onion.

7. After that, stir to break the onions apart and coat all the pieces with the oil.
8. In addition, cook, stirring occasionally, for about 5 minutes, or until the onions begin to brown.
9. After which you lower the heat to medium-low and continue to cook, stirring occasionally, for about 15 minutes, or until the onions are golden brown and quite crisp.
10. Then, using a slotted spoon, transfer the onions to a double layer of paper towels to drain. You can season with salt.
11. At this point, place the remaining tablespoon of oil in a large saucepan.
12. This is when you add the shallots and garlic and cook, stirring frequently, for about 5 minutes, or until just starting to color slightly.
13. After that, add the reserved greens along with the chopped herbs and cook, stirring, to heat through; taste and, if necessary, season with salt.

14. Finally, remove from the heat and transfer to a serving dish; drizzle with lemon juice and sprinkle the crisp onions over the top.
15. Make sure you serve immediately.

DELECTABLE BRAIN WASH DESSERTS

Favorite Chocolate Cake

Makes one 9-inch cake
Preparation Time: About 1¼ hours, + 4 or more hours for chilling

Tips:

1. **However, n**ot only is this cake flourless, it is also sugarless and also delicious, too.
2. This recipe does have to chill before cutting, so it is best made the day before you need to serve it. It will also make a great contribution to a bake sale, community event, or potluck dinner.

Ingredients:

Pinch of fine sea salt

⅔ cup of unsalted organic butter from grass-fed cows

Organic cocoa powder for dusting

5 large organic eggs from pasture-raised chickens, separated, at room temperature

9 ounces' organic dark chocolate, at least 80% cacao

2 teaspoons of pure organic vanilla extract

Directions:

1. Meanwhile, heat the oven to 325°F.
2. After which you generously butter the interior of a 9-inch round spring form pan.
3. After that, cut a parchment circle to fit the bottom of the pan and generously butter it as well.
4. At this point, place the egg whites in the bowl of an electric mixer fitted with a whisk attachment.
5. This is when you add the salt and beat on low speed until stiff peaks form; set aside.
6. Furthermore, place the chocolate and butter in the top half of a double boiler over boiling water and heat, stirring frequently, for about 4 minutes, or until the chocolate and butter have melted and combined.

7. After that, scrape the mixture into a large mixing bowl and, using a whisk, beat the egg yolks into the chocolate mixture one at a time.
8. Then, beat in the vanilla; gently fold in the egg whites, a bit at a time, until no white streaks remain.
9. In addition, pour the batter into the prepared pan and transfer to the preheated oven.
10. After which you bake for about an hour, or until the cake jiggles in the center but the outer edges are firm.
11. Then, you remove from the oven and set on a wire rack to cool; when cool, transfer to the refrigerator to set for at least 4 hours or overnight.
12. At this point, when ready to serve, unmold from the spring form pan, then pull off and discard the parchment paper.
13. Finally, place the cocoa powder in a fine-mesh sieve and gently tap to dust the top of the cake with cocoa.

BRAIN WASH RECIPES

14. You can cut into slices and serve.

Chocolate Chip Cookies

Makes about 2 dozen
Preparation Time: About 20 minutes
Tips:

1. I absolutely love the combination of almond flavors and chocolate in these cookies.
2. However, it is important that you use chocolate chips with at least 80% cacao; and if you toast the almonds, the cookies will have an even deeper almond flavor.
3. This recipe makes a great introduction to the Brain Wash diet.

Ingredients:
¼ cup of granulated organic stevia
¼ cup of organic coconut oil
½ cup of chopped raw unsalted organic almonds or walnuts
1¼ cups of organic almond flour
¼ teaspoon of baking soda
2 teaspoons of pure organic vanilla extract

½ cup of organic dark chocolate chips (at least 80% cacao)

Directions:

1. Meanwhile, heat the oven to 350°F.
2. After which you line two baking sheets with nonstick silicone liners or parchment paper.
3. After that, combine the stevia, almond flour, and baking soda in a medium mixing bowl.
4. Then, stir in the coconut oil and vanilla; when well combined, stir in the chocolate chips and nuts.
5. At this point, drop the dough by the heaping teaspoonful onto the prepared baking sheets.
6. This is when you transfer to the preheated oven and bake for about 9 minutes, or until set and golden around the edges.
7. Furthermore, remove from the oven and, using a spatula, transfer to wire racks to cool.

8. Finally, store in an airtight container at room temperature for no more than five days.

Almond-Coconut Biscotti

Makes 8 to 10

Preparation Time: 1 hour, plus 12 hours for resting if desired

Tip:

1. Remember, when you allow these biscotti to dry completely, they are great dunkers in an afternoon cup of tea.
2. This recipe can also be made without the stevia; they won't be sweet, but they will still be very satisfying.

Ingredients:

¼ cup of unsweetened organic coconut flakes

2 tablespoons of organic chia seeds

¼ cup of organic coconut oil

1 teaspoon of baking soda

2 cups of raw unsalted organic almonds

3 tablespoons of organic cocoa powder

1 large organic egg from a pasture-raised chicken (at room temperature)

1 tablespoon of granulated organic stevia

Directions:

1. First, combine the coconut, almonds, cocoa powder, and chia seeds in the bowl of a food processor fitted with a metal blade.
2. After which you pulse until the mixture resembles very fine crumbs.
3. After that, scrape the mixture into a medium mixing bowl.
4. Then, add the egg, stevia, coconut oil, and baking soda, beating to combine well.
5. Meanwhile, heat the oven to 375°F.
6. Furthermore, scrape the dough from the bowl and, using your hands, form it into a loaf about an inch thick.
7. At this point, wrap in plastic wrap and refrigerate for about 30 minutes, or until firmed slightly.
8. This is when you remove the dough from the refrigerator, unwrap, and cut crosswise into 8 to 10 bars of equal size.
9. In addition, lay the cookies about 1 inch apart on an ungreased cookie sheet. After

which you place in the preheated oven and bake for about 10 minutes, or until the dough has firmed somewhat and begun to color around the edges.

NOTE: you can either remove the cookies from the oven and serve them warm and soft or, for a crisper cookie, turn the oven off and let them stay in the cooling oven to dry slightly.

Remember, if you prefer very crisp biscotti, I suggest when the oven has cooled, remove the cookies and transfer to a wire rack to rest for 12 hours at room temperature.

Ricotta Mousse

Serves 4
Preparation Time: About 15 minutes
Tips:

1. This recipe is a light and refreshing dessert that can also be made with ½ cup of dark (at least 80% cacao) chocolate chips, alone or in combination with the berries.
2. Remember that this recipe travels well, so it is a terrific low-carb dessert to take to a potluck or a summer barbecue.

Ingredients:

¼ cup of organic heavy cream from grass-fed cows

¾ cup of organic blueberries or better still raspberries

Organic cocoa powder for dusting

2 cups of Ricotta Cheese

2 tablespoons of granulated organic stevia, or more to taste

1 teaspoon of freshly grated organic orange zest

Directions:

1. First, combine the Ricotta Cheese, cream, and stevia in the bowl of a food processor fitted with a metal blade and process until very light and smooth.
2. After which you scrape the mixture into a medium mixing bowl.
3. After that, gently stir in the berries and the orange zest.
4. Then, spoon an equal portion into each of four small dessert bowls.
5. Finally, dust with cocoa powder and serve.

NOTE: this recipe can be stored, covered and refrigerated, for a day or two.

Almond Panna Cotta

Serves 4 to 6

Preparation Time: About 30 minutes, + 4 hours or more for chilling

Tip:

This light dessert if you really want to fancy it up, I suggest you puree a cup of blueberries, spoon an equal portion of the puree on each serving plate, then garnish with whole berries and a mint leaf.

Ingredients:

1 cup of organic heavy cream from grass-fed cows (divided)

1 tablespoon of granulated organic stevia

4–6 organic mint leaves

1 cup of unsweetened organic almond milk

1½ teaspoons of unflavored gelatin

1 teaspoon of pure organic almond extract

½ cup of organic blueberries

Directions:

1. First, combine the almond milk with ½ cup of the heavy cream in a small heavy-bottom saucepan over low heat.
2. After which you heat for about 6 minutes, or until bubbles form around the edge of the pan.
3. Then, while the almond milk is heating, pour the remaining ½ cup of heavy cream into a medium heatproof mixing bowl.
4. After that, add the gelatin and let stand to soften.
5. Furthermore, when the almond milk mixture is hot, pour it over the gelatin mixture.
6. At this point, add the stevia and stir until completely blended; set aside to cool to room temperature.
7. Stir in the almond extract.
8. This is when you pour an equal portion of the mixture into either four 4-ounce ramekins or six smaller ramekins.

9. In addition, cover each ramekin with plastic wrap, and transfer to the refrigerator; let chill for at least 4 hours, or until firm.
10. If you want to serve, invert each ramekin onto a dessert plate.
11. After which you garnish with a few berries and a mint leaf.
12. Finally, if the panna cotta does not easily slip out of the ramekins, wrap the ramekins in a wet hot towel for a few seconds.
13. Make sure you serve immediately.

DRINKS

Matcha Smoothie

Serves 2
Preparation Time: About 5 minutes
Tip:

1. This recipe is a wonderful afternoon energy booster—refreshing, delectable, and so good for you.
2. Feel free to add a couple of ice cubes to it while blending for a bit of slushiness in the final drink.

Ingredients:
¼ cup of organic mint leaves
2 cups of chilled organic coconut water
2 large organic Persian cucumbers
½ teaspoon of organic matcha (green tea powder)
Directions:

1. First, chop the cucumbers and place them in a blender.
2. After which you add the mint leaves, matcha, and coconut water and process until very smooth.
3. Finally, pour into two glasses and serve.

Afternoon Pick-Me-Up

Serves 2
Preparation Time: About 7 minutes
Tips:

1. This drink is just the perfect thing to wake you up in the late afternoon.
2. Remember, if you've limited your carbs during the day, you might splurge and add half a small banana for a little more texture and sweetness; but if you do, remember to keep the remainder of your carb intake low.

Ingredients:

2 cups of chopped trimmed organic kale leaves
1 cup of chilled organic unsweetened almond milk
1 teaspoon of freshly squeezed organic lime juice
1 organic avocado (peeled and seeded)
1 cup of chilled organic coconut water
2 tablespoons of chopped organic mint leaves
1 tablespoon of chopped organic ginger

Directions:

1. First, combine all ingredients in a blender.
2. After which you process until smooth and creamy.
3. After that, place a few ice cubes in each of two large glasses and divide the mixture between the two.
4. Make sure you serve immediately.

Hibiscus Tea

Serves 4

Preparation Time: About 15 minutes
Tips:

1. However, hot or iced hibiscus tea is frequently the beverage of choice for people who are fasting.
2. I cherish its fruitiness and its ability to refresh on a hot summer day.
3. Remember, ginger and herbs seem to be great partners for this wonderfully healing tea.

Ingredients:
7 organic basil leaves
1 tablespoon of freshly squeezed organic lime juice
4 organic mint sprigs for garnish (it is optional)
⅓ cup of dried organic hibiscus flowers
½-inch knob organic ginger (peeled)
Granulated organic stevia to taste (it is optional)

Directions:

1. First, combine the hibiscus flowers, ginger, basil, and 4 cups cold water in a medium saucepan.
2. After which you place over medium heat and bring to a boil.
3. After that, immediately remove from the heat, cover, and set aside to steep for 15 minutes.
4. Then, stir in the lime juice and, if using, the stevia.
5. At this point, strain into a teapot or, if serving chilled, a pitcher.

NOTE: if the latter, either add ice or refrigerate for a couple of hours to chill.

6. Furthermore, serve garnished with a mint sprig if desired.

NOTE: you can use fresh organically grown hibiscus flowers if it is available instead of dried leaves to make the tea.

7. Finally, remove the green part at the base of the flower along with the pistil (the thin thread in the center that holds the pollen) and proceed just as you would with dried leaves.

Gingerade

Makes about 2 quarts
Preparation Time: About 40 minutes
Tips:

1. This is an old recipe that was used as a pick-me-up during times of hot, hard farm work.
2. However, it should not be sweet; the refreshing tang of ginger is what serves to revitalize and refresh.
3. Remember, it is a delicious drink to serve at backyard parties and beach picnics.

Ingredients:
Peel of 3 organic lemons (cut into thin strips)
Juice of 3 organic lemons
Organic mint sprigs for garnish (it is optional)
6 ounces' organic ginger (peeled and chopped)
Peel of 1 organic orange (cut into thin strips)
Juice of one organic orange
Granulated organic stevia (to taste)

Directions:

1. First, combine the ginger with the citrus peels in a large saucepan.
2. After which you pour 2 quarts of boiling water over the mixture, cover, and set aside to steep for 30 minutes, or until the liquid is very fragrant.
3. After that, add the citrus juice and the stevia, stirring to blend.
4. Then, add only a tiny bit of the stevia at a time and taste after each addition. **NOTE:** the beverage should be quite gingery and tart.
5. Finally, when ready to serve, fill a large pitcher with ice and pour the gingerade over it.

Remember, if you so desire, place a mint sprig in each glass as you serve.

Powerhouse Coffee

Serves 2

Preparation Time: About 5 minutes

Tips:

1. Remember, this coffee drink can start your day off with a bang or end it with a sizzle.
2. However, it is rather like a delicious, rich cappuccino that turns into an enticing dessert.
3. I suggest you make use of a high-speed blender such as a Vitamix so that all the ingredients emulsify into a creamy mixture.

Ingredients:

3 tablespoons of finely grated organic dark chocolate, at least 80% cacao

1 tablespoon of MCT oil

Organic ground cinnamon (for garnish)

2 cups of hot strong brewed organic coffee

2 tablespoons of organic unsalted butter from grass-fed cows, at room temperature

2 tablespoons of organic heavy cream from grass-fed cows

Directions:

1. First, combine the coffee, butter, chocolate, and oil in a high-speed blender.
2. After which you process for a minute or so, or until the mixture is smooth and creamy.
3. After that, pour into two warmed coffee cups, then spoon 1 tablespoon of heavy cream into each cup and sprinkle with ground cinnamon.
4. Then, serve immediately.

Turmeric Milk Shake

Serves 2
Preparation Time: About 7 minutes
Tips:

1. This recipe is best made with fresh turmeric and ginger in a high-speed blender such as a Vitamix.
2. Make sure you grate the turmeric and ginger to ensure that the finished drink will be smooth and creamy.
3. Feel free to use almond milk and coconut oil in place of the coconut milk and avocado oil.
4. Remember, if you have fresh coconut, it will add a lovely flavor, though it's not necessary.

Ingredients:

2 tablespoons of organic avocado oil
1-inch piece of organic ginger, peeled and grated, or 1 teaspoon organic ground ginger
1 teaspoon of pure organic vanilla extract

4 ice cubes

3¼ cups of organic unsweetened coconut milk (chilled)

5-inch piece fresh organic turmeric root, peeled and grated, or 2 teaspoons of organic ground turmeric

¼ cup of unsweetened shredded or better still flaked organic coconut

1 teaspoon of freshly grated organic orange zest, + more for garnish

½ teaspoon of organic ground cinnamon

Directions:

1. First, combine the coconut milk and avocado oil in the jar of a high-speed blender.
2. After which you process to just blend.
3. After that, add the ginger, vanilla, turmeric, coconut, orange zest, and cinnamon and process to just combine.
4. Then, add the ice cubes and process on high until the mixture is smooth, thick, and bright yellow.

5. Furthermore, pour an equal portion into each of two tall glasses.
6. Finally, sprinkle the top with orange zest and serve.

www.ingramcontent.com/pod-product-compliance
Lightning Source LLC
Chambersburg PA
CBHW012100090526
44592CB00017B/2639